YOUR KNOWLEDGE HAS VALUE

AF130177

- We will publish your bachelor's and
  master's thesis, essays and papers

- Your own eBook and book -
  sold worldwide in all relevant shops

- Earn money with each sale

Upload your text at www.GRIN.com
and publish for free

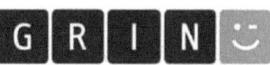

Bibliographic information published by the German National Library:

The German National Library lists this publication in the National Bibliography; detailed bibliographic data are available on the Internet at http://dnb.dnb.de .

Imprint:

Copyright © 2016 GRIN Verlag
Print and binding: Books on Demand GmbH, Norderstedt Germany
ISBN: 9783668275645

This book at GRIN:

https://www.grin.com/document/336144

Wakjira Kebede, Kibeb Legese, Jaleta Shuka

Isolation and identification of the Newcastle disease virus

GRIN Verlag

GRIN - Your knowledge has value

Since its foundation in 1998, GRIN has specialized in publishing academic texts by students, college teachers and other academics as e-book and printed book. The website www.grin.com is an ideal platform for presenting term papers, final papers, scientific essays, dissertations and specialist books.

Visit us on the internet:

http://www.grin.com/

http://www.facebook.com/grincom

http://www.twitter.com/grin_com

ADDIS ABABA UNIVERSITY

COLLEGE OF VETERINARY MEDICINE AND AGRICULTURE

ISOLATION AND IDENTIFICATION OF NEWCASTLE DISEASE VIRUS

BY:

WAKJIRA KEBEDE DABA

A TERM PAPER SUBMITTED TO COLLEGE OF VETERINARY MEDICINE AND
AGRICULTURE, ADDIS ABABA UNIVERSITY, IN PARTIAL FULFILLMENT FOR
THE ATTAINMENT OF THE BSC DEGREE IN VETERINARY LABORATORY
TECHNOLOGY

MAY, 2016

BISHOFTU, ETHIOPIA

ACKNOWLEDGEMENTS

First of all, I wish to express my sincere gratitude to my advisor Dr. Kibeb Legese and Dr. Jaleta Shuka for their valuable advice, guidance and constructive comments in directing and shaping the research idea.

I am also indebted to National Veterinary Institute (NVI) and its management who provided me this opportunity to attend this program.

I would like to thank staff members of Ada district veterinary clinic Dr. Tsigie G/Michael, Ato Belay Temesgen and Ato Efirem shimelis, who helped me during clinical examination and sample collection.

My appreciation also goes to W/ro Berhan Demeke who helped me during the period of laboratory analysis and for her constructive comments.

Last but not least, my colleagues at NVI helped me a lot; especially Dr. Hundera Sori, Ato Kasaye Adamu for their help during laboratory works.

Contents

ACKNOWLEDGEMENTS 2

Contents 3

LIST OF ABBREVIATION... 4

LIST OF TABLES 5

LIST OF FIGURES 6

SUMMARY 7

1. INTRODUCTION 8

2. METHOD OF CLINICAL DATA COLLECTION 9

    2.1. Study area.. 9

    2.2. Study animal 9

    2.3. Case report 9

    2.4. Clinical Examination 9

    2.5. Sample collection 10

3. LABORATORY ANALYSIS... 10

    3.1. Sample processing and storage.. 10

    3.2. Virus isolation 10

        3.2.1. Haemagglutination test (HA).. 12

        3.2.2. Haemagglutination test results 12

    3.3. Virus identification 13

        3.3.1. Haemagglutination inhibition test (HI).. 13

4. RESULT AND DISCUSSION 14

    4.1. Clinical Diagnosis 14

    4.2. Virus isolation 14

    4.3. Virus identification 15

5. CONCLUSION AND RECOMMENDATION 16

6. REFERENCES 17

7.APPENDIXES.. 18

LIST OF ABBREVIATION

APMV	**Avian paramixo virus**
AB	**Anti body**
APMV	**Avian paramixo virus**
^{0}c	**Degree celcious**
cRBC	**Chicken red blood cell**
FAO	**Food and agricultural organization**
HA	**Haemagglutination**
HAU	**Haemagglutination unit**
HB1	**Vaccinal strain for Newcastle virus**
HI	**Haemagglutination inhibition**
ML	**Mili liter**
NCD	**Newcastle disease**
NCDV	**Newcastle disease virus**
NVI	**National Veterinary Institute**
OIE	**Office Des International Epizootics**
PBS	**Phosphate buffered saline**
PCV	**Packed cell volume**
RBCS	**Red blood cells**
RPM	**Revolution per minute**
SPF	**Specific pathogenic free**
µl	**Micro liter**

LIST OF TABLES

Table 1. Result of history and clinical examination

Table 2. Result of virus isolated using NCD virus antibody free specific embryonated eggs

Table 3. Haemagglutination inhibition test of collected serum

LIST OF FIGURES

Figure 1. SPF eggs for inoculation

Figure 2. Incubated SPF eggs

Figure 3. Inoculated and ceiled eggs

Figure 4. Candling eggs

Figure 5. Harvesting of allantoic fluid

Figure 6.RBC and different materials used for test

Figure 7. Micro haemagglutination test in a v- bottomed micro plate

Figure 8. Haemagglutination inhibition test on micro plate

SUMMARY

Newcastle disease (NCD) is a contagious bird disease affecting domestic and wild avian species characterised by respiratory signs (gasping, coughing, nervous signs depression, in appetence, muscular tremors, and drooping wings, twisting of head and neck, greenish watery diarrhoea, misshapen, rough-or thin shelled eggs and reduced egg production. This study was designed for isolation and identification of Newcastle disease virus from sick and suspected chicken in poultry farm, Bishoftu, Ethiopia, during October 16, 20015- May 30, 2016 which brought to research and diagnostic laboratory in National Veterinary Institute (NVI), Ethiopia by owner. Total suspected chicken were 200 and out of these 30 chickens were brought to NVI and samples were collected. The sample included serum, cloacal and tracheal swab. Serum sample was collected for confirmatory diagnosis by serological HI test. HI result has showed that more than 80% of the total samples collected were positive for Newcastle disease virus (NCDV). Isolation of the virus from cloacal and tracheal swabs was performed by inoculating each suspected sample in to 10 day old embryonating eggs. Out of 30 NCDV suspected samples 24 (6 layers and 18 broilers) were positive for NCD virus isolation. Out of the 24 HA positive NCD virus suspected samples 24(6 layers and 18broilers were HI positive.

Keywords:- Newcastle disease virus, isolation,Haemagglutination, Haemagglutination inhibition.

1. INTRODUCTION

Newcastle disease (NCD) is a highly contagious and often severe disease found worldwide that affects birds including domestic poultry. It is caused by a virus in the family of paramyxoviruses. The disease appears in three forms: lentogenic or mild, mesogenic or moderate and velogenic or very virulent, also called exotic Newcastle disease. The lentogenic strains are very widespread, but cause few disease outbreaks. It usually presents as a respiratory disease, but depression, nervous manifestations, or diarrhea may be the predominant clinical form. NCD, in its highly pathogenic form, is a disease listed in the World Organization for Animal Health (OIE) Terrestrial Animal Health Code and must be reported to the OIE (OIE Terrestrial Animal Health Code. 2010).

The poultry sector of Ethiopia is mainly based on chicken production and concerned with egg and meat requirements. The total chicken in the country is estimated to be about 58 million of which 95.87%, 3.6% and 0.53% were reported to be indigenous, hybrid and exotic breeds, respectively (CSA,2 008; Ashanafi, 2000). The chicken kept under traditional or "back yard" conditions accounts for 99%, while only 1% birds are rearing under intensive management system in commercial farms (CSA; Almargot, 1987).

Despite of large number of chicken, the benefit of chicken contribution to the country is far away from the existing potentials. This is because of inadequate feed supply, improper production system, and high prevalence of disease, poor animal genetic resources and poor marketing (Alemu, 2010). Among those disease affects poultry Newcastle disease is one of poultry disease inflicting heavy loss in Ethiopia. The disease has a local name *"Fengel"*which literary mean collapsing (Ashanafi, 2000).

Bio-security and vaccination are two important measures for prevention and control the disease in the country and have been successful where the measures are properly implemented. However, there both measures have mostly been used in commercial intensive and semi-intensive production systems of the country. This gap makes the disease prevalent in backyard production system. According to work done by Ashenafi (2000) some farmers have given up rearing poultry because of disease problem.

There have been several cases of the Newcastle disease come to NVI for diagnosis from nearby areas. Virus isolation, haemaglutination test and Serological diagnosis test are most utilized to diagnose the disease. However, serological test is necessary to confirm the disease since haemagglutination has its own drawback.

Therefore, the objective of this study is:

- ➤ To isolate and identify Newcastle disease virus from cases brought to national veterinary institute diagnostic laboratory
- ➤ To determine NCD virus strain present in the Bishoftu town
- ➤ To forward prevention methods to the stoke holders

2. METHOD OF CLINICAL DATA COLLECTION

2.1. Study area

Accordingly, clinical materials (serum, tracheal and cloacl swab) were collected from NCD suspected chicken reared under semi-intensive poultry farm located at Bishoftu town which was located at distance of 47km to the south east of Addis Ababa. The area is situated at latitude of 09^0 and longitude of 04^0 and has elevation of 1850m above sea level. The mean minimum and maximum temperature of the town ranges from 12.3^0c to 27.7^0c with an average annual rain fall of 800 mm and mean relative humidity of 61.3% *(CSA, 2001)*.

2.2. Study animal

From total 200 clinically sick exotic breeds chicken samples were collected from 30 highly sick chickens (20 broilers and 10 layers) which were in different ages (3weeks-6months). The chickens were come from one farm found in Bishoftu. According to the information obtained from the owner, all chickens were reared under semi-intensive farming.

2.3. Case report

Owner was brought his clinically sick chickens after one to two days of the commencement of the disease. Loss of appetite, depression, diarrhea, inability to stand, swelling of comb and wattle, nasal and eye discharge and reduction of egg yield were the main symptoms which were explained by the owner. The owner also indicated the presence of death of some chickens after they had showed the similar signs. Moreover, the owner responded that his flocks were not vaccinated against NCD.

2.4. Clinical Examination

Clinical examination was made based on history the owner of the farm complained. Based on inspection, the sick chickens had showed depression, weakness paralysis of legs and wings, dehydration, edema of the head and wattles, difficulty in breathing were the main clinical signs observed during inspection.

2.5. Sample collection

Samples were collected, transported and stored according to (OIE.2010) protocol. Out of 200 clinically sick chickens, cloacal and tracheal swabs were collected from 30 chickens which were tentatively diagnosed as highly infected by NCD and selected for sample collection. The samples were collected by using sterile cotton swab. Each sample was placed in labeled screw cap test tube having isotonic phosphate buffered saline (PBS), PH 7.2 – 7.4, containing antibiotics. The blood serum of bird had also collected for inhibition test. (OIE, 2012)

3. LABORATORY ANALYSIS

3.1. Sample processing and storage

Standard sample storage and processing for NCDV test was employed (OIE, 2012). Each cloacal and tracheal sample was centrifuged at 2500rpm for 10 minutes to obtain clarified supernatant suspension of test virus at temperature not exceeding 25^0c by using labeled test tube having isotonic phosphate buffered saline (PBS), pH 7.0–7.4, containing antibiotics and stored at $+4^0c$ until viral isolation.

3.2. Virus isolation

Incubated eggs were candled and eggs which have viable embryo selected and marked on air space for inoculation. Marked eggs were disinfected with 70% ethanol. The supernatant fluid expected to contain the virus was inoculated in 0.2 ml volumes into the allantoic cavity of 10 day embryonated SPF fowl eggs. After inoculation, it was incubated at 37°C for 7 days. Candling was carried out every 24 hours during incubation period of the infected embryonated eggs. Eggs containing dead or dying embryos as they arose, and all eggs remaining at the end of the incubation period was chilled to 4°C for overnight and then allantoic fluid was harvested.

The harvested allantioc fluid from each egg was checked for haemagglutination activity (OIE, 2012) and the remaining harvested allantoic fluid was kept at -20^{0}c for further study.

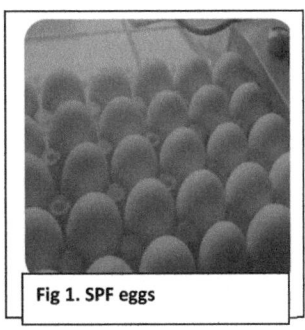

Fig 1. SPF eggs

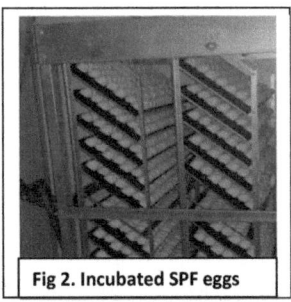

Fig 2. Incubated SPF eggs

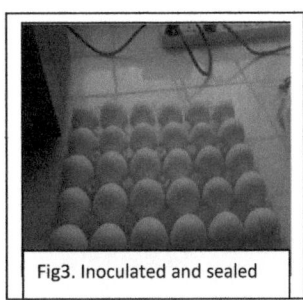

Fig3. Inoculated and sealed

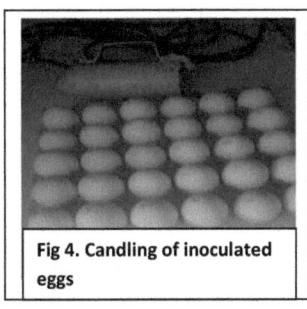

Fig 4. Candling of inoculated eggs

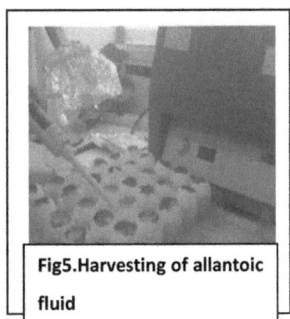

Fig5.Harvesting of allantoic fluid

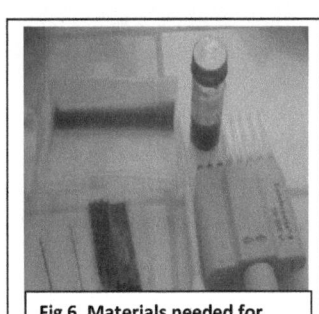

Fig 6. Materials needed for test

3.2.1. Haemagglutination test (HA)

This test was conducted to confirm the presence of NCD virus in the allantoic fluid of eggs inoculated with supernatant fluid which got from samples.50 μL of allantoic fluid from each eggs was taken and placed each drop in a separate well of "V" shaped microtitre plate.25 μL of 1% fowl red blood cell was added to each well that had allantoic fluid and mixed gently. This kept at room temperature for 45 minutes and read the result.

3.2.2. Haemagglutination test results

- ✓ Agglutinated red blood cells in suspension have a clumped appearance distinct from non-agglutinated red blood cells.
- ✓ The red blood cells mixed with the positive control allantoic fluid will clump within one minute.
- ✓ The red blood cells mixed with the PBS and negative control allantoic fluid remain as an even suspension and do not clump. Judge the results of the test sample by comparison with the positive and negative controls.

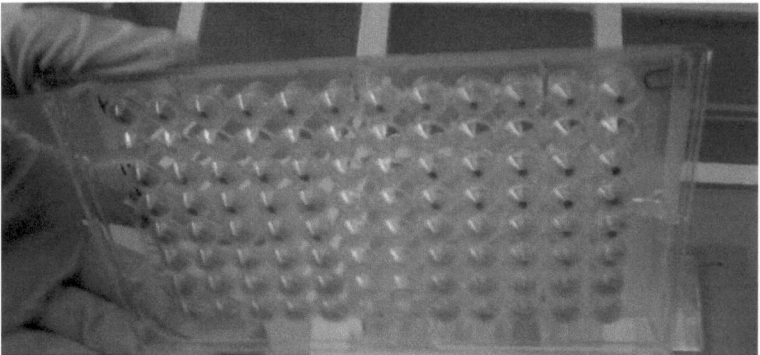

Fig.7. Micro haemagglutination test in a V-bottome microwell plate

3.3. Virus identification

3.3.1. Haemagglutination inhibition test (HI)

To perform HI test, 4 Haemagglutination units (4HA units) was prepared for working antigen. This known antigen was obtained from National Veterinary Institute (NVI), Ethiopia. (The procedure to prepare 4HA is written in Appendix 1.4.). Each blood serum collected from sick chicken was tested for the presence of antibody of NCD virus. 25 µL PBS was dispensed in to each well of a 96-well V-bottomed microtitre plate. After shaking a test serum, 25 µL of serum added to the first and the last (control) well of each row. By using multichannel pipetter, made serial two fold dilutions of each serum sample along the row by transferring 25 µL of fluid from one well to the next stopped at the second last well. 25 µL of fluid from the second last well of the row was discarded. The last well of each well did not diluted (control).Then 25 µL of 4 HA units added to each well except control well. Mixed the well gently, covered and kept at room temperature for 30 minutes. Then after 25 µL of 1%suspension of red blood cell added to each well and tapped gently the side of plate to mix and cover and kept at room temperature for 45 minutes and read the result.

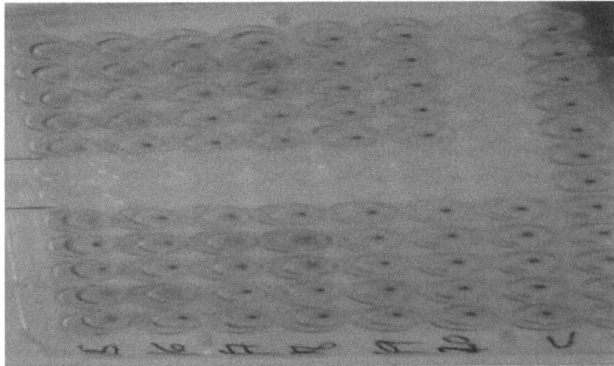

Fig. 8. Haemagglutination inhibition test on micro plate

4. RESULT AND DISCUSSION

4.1. Clinical Diagnosis

Clinically, 18(90%) birds of 20 layers chickens and 7(70%) of 10 affected broilers were diagnosed as Newcastle (Table 1) which means 83.33% were suspected. The most clinical signs observed were depression, edema of the head and wattle, twisted neck and paralysis, loss of weight and greenish diarrhea.

Table1. Result of history and clinical examination

Total	no,	of	No, of suspected chickens for NCD			Prevalence (%)		
Broilers	*Layers*	*Broilers*	*Layers*	*Total*		*Broilers*	*Layers*	**Total**
20	10	18	17	25		60	23.33	83.33

4.2. Virus isolation

A total of 24(90%) samples for 30 clinically diagnosed Newcastle affected chickens, were positive for virus isolation in embryonated eggs (table 2). In all positive cases embryo died within 72 - 168 hours of post inoculation. All of 24 samples showed positive to HA activity which indicate that the isolate were heamagulitinating virus.

Table2. Result of virus isolated using NCD virus antibody free specific embryonated eggs

No, of samples inoculated			*No, of positivechickens for NCD*			*percentage (%)*
Broilers	*Layers*	*Total*	*Broilers*	*Layers*	*Total*	
20	10	30	18	6	24	80

4.3. Virus identification

All 25 tested serum showed settled red blood cell in the bottom of well (Figure) and HI result of total sample found in range of 16:128 (Table 3). This amount range showed the chicken is infected with ND virus.

Table 3. Hemaglutination inhibition test result of collected serum

Sample code	sample type	HI titer result	Interpretation
S1	Serum	1:16	Positive NDV
S2	Serum	1:32	Positive NDV
S3	Serum	1:128	Positive NDV
S4	Serum	1:32	Positive NDV
S5	Serum	1:64	Positive NDV
S6	Serum	1:64	Positive NDV
S7	Serum	1:32	Positive NDV
S8	Serum	1:64	Positive NDV
S9	Serum	1:128	Positive NDV
S10	Serum	1:128	Positive NDV
S11	Serum	1:64	Positive NDV
S12	Serum	1:32	Positive NDV
S13	Serum	1:64	Positive NDV
S14	Serum	1:32	Positive NDV
S15	Serum	1:32	Positive NDV
S16	Serum	1:64	Positive NDV
S17	Serum	1:64	Positive NDV
S18	Serum	1:128	Positive NDV
S19	Serum	1:64	Positive NDV
S20	Serum	1:128	Positive NDV
S21	Serum	1:64	Positive NDV
S22	Serum	1:64	Positive NDV
S23	Serum	1:32	Positive NDV
S24	Serum	1:128	Positive NDV

5. CONCLUSION AND RECOMMENDATION

In this study the presence of NCD virus in chickens coming from poultry farm was confirmed based on clinical signs, virus isolation and identification.

The prevalence of ND in poultry farms of the country should be taken as a potential threat for the poultry industry. As ND is viral disease, no specific treatment is effective after infection. Therefore, practicing preventive strategies is the only mechanism to control the disease.

Based on the above conclusion the following recommendations are forwarded
- ✓ The vaccine should be availed through local production by the NVI and vaccination of all the chicken at risk age group.
- ✓ Training and awareness creation about the disease should be made to all stockholders' of the sector including farmers.
- ✓ Effort must be done to study how to minimize the disease incidence to improve productivity and to eliminate the disease from the country.

6. REFERENCES

Alemu, (2010): Drug Administration and control authority of Ethiopia, (2006): standard treatment guidelines for veterinary practice, 1st edition. Addis Ababa Ethiopia.

Alexander DJ (2003): Newcastle disease, other avian paramyxoviruses, and pneumoviru Infections. *In*: Saif Y, Barnes JH

Alexander DJ,(2001):Newcastle disease- the Golden Memorial lecture Britain veterinary science, 42,5-22.

CSA, 2008; Almargot, 1987: avian pathology of industrial farms in Ethiopia. In IAR proceed ings, First National livestock improvement conference, Addis Ababa agricultural research institute, Ethiopia. Pp 114-117.

CSA,2008; Ashenafi ,H. (2000): survey on identifications of major disease of local chickens in three selected agro climatic zone in central Ethiopia. DVM thesis, Faculty of veterinary medicine, Addis Ababa University, Debre Zeit, Ethiopia.

CSA, 2001: statics agency report, Addis Ababa Ethiopia

NVI, (1974): Poultry disease and Newcastle disease record book, Debre Zeit, Ethiopia.

OIE (2012): Manual of diagnostic test and vaccine for terrestrial animals, version adopted by world assembly delegate in may.

OIE (2012): Manual of diagnostic test and vaccine for terrestrial animals, adopted may 2012, 6thed. Office international des epizootics. Paris, France. World assembly delegate in May.

Tadelle, D. (1996): Studies on village poultry production system in central high lands of Wilson, Ethiopia. Msc thesis, university of Uppsala, Sweden.

7.APPENDIXES

Annex.1. Materials and reagent required
- ✓ Water bath, incubator, and vortex
- ✓ V-bottomed micro titre plates
- ✓ Single channel micropipettes
- ✓ Fowl RBC(ARBC)
- ✓ Trough
- ✓ Syringe
- ✓ PBS buffer at PH 7.2 – 7.4
- ✓ Elsevier's solution
- ✓ NCD virus antigen
- ✓ Positive and negative control
- ✓ Bi-distilled water
- ✓ Arranged test sera sheets of plate lay out

Annex.2. Reagent preparation

1. **Phosphate buffered saline (PBS) without calcium or magnesium**

✓ Sodium chloride	8.0g
✓ Potassium chloride	0.2g
✓ Potassium dihydrogen orthophosphate	0.2g
✓ Disodium hydrogen orthophosphate	1.44g
✓ Distilled water	1000ml
✓ Sterilized by Autoclave	

2. **70% ethanol alcohol**

Mix 70ml of absolute ethanol (100%) with 30ml distilled water

3. Preparing a washed red blood cell suspension

➤ Measure the required volume of anticoagulant into a sterile screw-capped bottle or centrifuge tube. Use equal volumes of Alsever's solution and blood.

➤ Draw the anticoagulant (Alsever's solution or ACD) into a 10 mL syringe.

➤ Collect blood from one donor chicken. Gently mix the blood and anticoagulant in the syringe.

➤ Remove the needle and discharge the blood into the bottle or centrifuge tube containing anticoagulant. Roll gently to mix the blood.

➤ Collect blood from the remaining donor chickens (repeat steps 3 and 4 for each chicken).

➤ Fill the bottle with PBS and mix gently.

➤ Centrifuge at 1500 rpm for 10 minutes to sediment the red blood cells.

➤ Remove the supernatant using a Pasteur pipette and discard. Do not disturb the red blood cell layer at the base.

➤ Refill the bottle or centrifuge tube with PBS.

➤ Mix gently to resuspend the cells and centrifuge again for 10 minutes at 1500 rpm. Rough mixing may cause haemolysis of the red cells.

➤ Remove the supernatant using a Pasteur pipette and discard.

➤ Refill the centrifuge tube with PBS.

➤ Mix gently to resuspend the cells.

➤ Pour the blood into 10ml calibrated centrifuge tubes and centrifuge again for 10 minutes at 1500 rpm.

➤ Remove the supernatant using a Pasteur pipette and discard,

➤ Measure the volume of the red blood cell layer using the graduations on the wall of the centrifuge tube.

➤ Add PBS to the red blood cell layer to make a final 10% red blood cell suspension. For example, if the volume of the red blood cell layer is 1ml, add 9 ml PBS to make a total volume of 10 ml.

➤ Mix gently to resuspend the cells, transfer the red blood cell suspension to a screw - capped bottle, label and store at 4^0C.

4. Preparation of 4 HA units of ND virus antigen suspension

❖ Using the quantitative HA test, titrate the ND virus antigen suspensions and calculate the HA titer.

❖ Divide the HA titer by four to calculate the dilution factor.

❖ Calculate the volume of diluted antigen suspension required. Allow 2.5 ml for each micro-titer plate.

❖ Measure the volume of antigen suspension required and dilute in PBS

5. NCD virus antigen titration

✓ Dispense 50μl of PBS in each micro plate.

✓ Add 50μl of known NCDV antigen in to each well.

✓ Add 50μl of 1% ARBC suspension in all wells & shake the plate &let it stay 30 minutes at room temperature.

✓ The last well where there is agglutination represents the dilution having one haemagglutinatin unit (HAU) per 50 μl

✓ Adjust your antigen to 4-8HAU 50 μl

6. The proper hem agglutination test (OIE, 2012)

⬇ Before testing, the sera are treated in a water bath at 58^0c for 30 minutes.

⬇ Make two fold test serum dilution at avolumes of 25 μl

⬇ Add 4-8 HAU 25 μl antigens in each well.

⬇ Shake plate and keep for 15minutes at room temperature.

⬇ Finally add 50 μl of a 1% RBC suspension. Shake it well and let it stay for 30 minutes.

⬇ *Interpretation:-* The last dilution where there is complete inhibition of haemagglutination represents the titration of the serum. the of point of NCDV is 1:16, so the sample which has the last dilution ≥ 1:16 are positive.

7. Haemagglutination inhibition test procedure (OIE, 2012)

- 25 μl of PBS was dispensed in to each well of a plastic V-bottomed micro titre plate.
- 25 μl of chicken anti-sera was placed in first well of the plate.
- Two fold dilution of 25 μl volumes of the serum made across the plate.
- 4HAU virus/antigen 25 μl is added in each well and the plate is left for minimum of 30minutes at room temperature.
- 25 μl of 1%(v/v)chicken RBCs is added to each well and after gentle mixing, the RBCs are allowed to settle for about 40minutes at a room temperature.
- The HAI titre is highest dilution of serum causing complete inhibition of 4HAU of antigen. The agglutination is assessed by tilting the plate. Only those wells in which the RBCs stream at the same rate as control wells (positive serum, virus/antigen and PBS control) was considered to show inhibition.
- The validity of result should assess against a negative control serum which should not give a titre greater than ¼ and positive control serum for which the titre was within dilution of known titre. HAI regarded as being positive if there was inhibition at antigen dilution 1/16 or more against 4HAU.

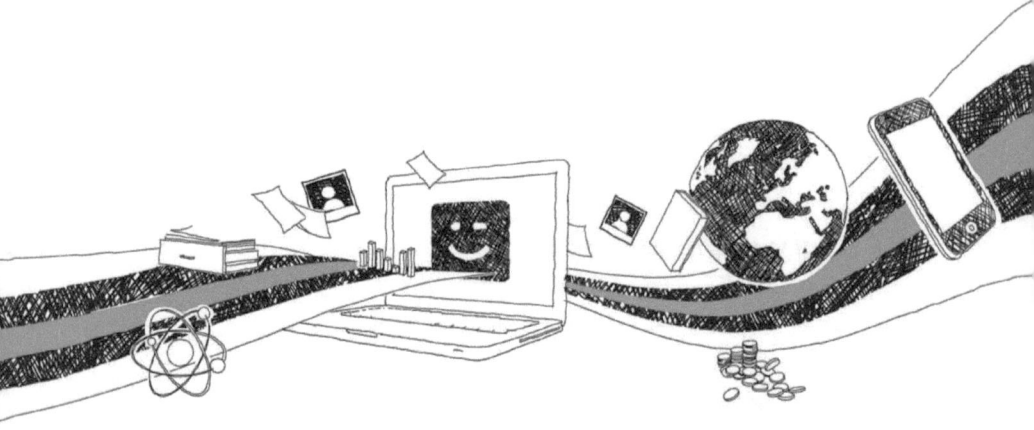
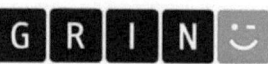